Lose weight and live a healthy life:

A simple guide to lose weight for men and women:

Sam Davis

Table of Contents

Chapter 1

Behaviors that help lose weight

Habits for a healthy decrease of weight.

It can be difficult to lose weight, and there are many different theories on how to achieve it.

The basic truth is that when it comes to weight loss, "one size does not fit all." Age, sex, body shape, underlying diseases, physical activity, genetics, prior dieting experiences, and even food preferences are all fundamental variables that might affect a person's capacity to lose weight and keep it off.

Even though there isn't one "ideal" diet for weight reduction. Avoiding a sedentary lifestyle, avoiding soda, and emphasizing food quality rather than calorie count are a few of them.

Here are habits that might help with weight reduction and healthy eating efforts:

1. Be aware of your starting point. For three days, note what you eat. Keep a record of the portions you consume as well as the entire menu you consume. Determine how frequently you dine out, order takeout, or buy meals on the go.

2. Specify your objective and create a plan. What is the aim? Do you wish to get healthier by losing weight? Do you wish you could squeeze into a worn-out pair of jeans? How will you accomplish your objective? Plan to prepare more meals at home? Will you consume fewer servings? Be specific and take baby steps.

3. Identify obstacles to your goals and devise strategies to get through them. Could having a full schedule prevent me from going to the gym? Obtain an hour's head start. Has a bare pantry kept you from preparing meals

at home? Look for some nutritious recipes, and then go to the shop prepared by writing down the goods you'll need.

4. Recognize your present eating behaviors that are unhealthy. Do you eat snacks in front of the TV to unwind and treat yourself? Do you miss lunch only to get ravenous by midday and eager to devour whatever you come across? When you begin to feel full, do you still eat everything on your plate?

5. Manage your portion sizes. Refresh your memory of typical serving sizes. Did you know that a serving of meat or poultry weighs 4 ounces, or the same amount as a deck of cards? or that there is only 1/2 cup of pasta in a serving?

6. Recognize satiety and hunger cues. Know the difference between bodily and emotional hunger. Do you eat when your body physically responds to food in some way? Or do you eat when you're nervous, depressed,

bored, or stressed? Try to stop eating BEFORE you feel full since it takes your brain 20 minutes to process signals from your stomach telling you to stop. High-fiber meals including vegetables, whole grains, beans, legumes, protein (fish, poultry, eggs), and water are foods that can make you feel more satisfied.

7. Pay attention to the improvements. It usually takes three months or longer to change behavior. Even if you make mistakes along the road, keep going. Obtain assistance from others and give yourself time to recognize the improvements you have made.

8. Put your entire health first. Find things you like and do them every day, whether it be walking, dancing, biking, raking leaves, or gardening. Instead of focusing on "diet" foods, choose seasonal, whole, high-quality foods.

9. Take your time and eat gently. Enjoy your meal from start to finish. Spend some time savoring the flavors, textures, and scents of the food you are eating.It requires time and effort to change habits. Your health will improve if you make a few minor changes now.

Beyond losing weight there is a need to manage your weight:Some of these ideas can be very beneficial

Ideas for changing behavior to manage weight

Adopting a healthy lifestyle that includes knowledge of nutrition and exercise, a good outlook, and the appropriate level of motivation is necessary for weight management.

Your odds of long-term weight management success are raised by internal factors including improved health, more energy, self-worth, and self-control.

Keep in mind to set reasonable goals and consider long-term success. You can achieve it if you believe in yourself. You can get inspiration from the following material to help you achieve your objectives.

Control the Environment in Your Home

Only eat at the kitchen or dining room table when seated.

Eat nothing when working on the internet, reading, cooking, chatting on the phone, or standing in front of the refrigerator.

Don't buy enticing meals; keep them away from the house.

Keep all enticing foods hidden. Have low-calorie foods accessible.

Keep out of the kitchen unless you are cooking.

Have low-fat string cheese, nonfat cottage cheese, tiny pieces of fruit, veggies, canned fruit, pretzels, and other healthful snacks on hand.

Take Control of Your Workplace

Avoid eating at your workstation and avoid leaving enticing treats there.

Plan nutritious snacks and bring them to work if you are hungry between meals.

Instead of eating during your breaks, go for a stroll.

Plan the one thing you'll eat at meals if you work around food. Make it uncomfortable to eat by chewing gum, eating sugarless candies, or sipping water or another calorie-free liquid.

Avoid working during meals. Meal skipping slows metabolism and may cause overeating at the following meal.

If food is served on special occasions, choose the healthiest option, munch on low-fat snacks brought from home, refuse all food, select one dish and eat a limited quantity, or stick to drinks.

Take Charge of the Dining Environment

Serve your meal at the kitchen counter or stove.

Keep the serving utensils off the table. If you do place dishes on the table, take them off as soon as you are done eating.

Your dish should be half veggies, quarter lean protein, and quarter carbohydrate.

Use smaller dishes, cups, and plates. In a tiny dish, a smaller piece will appear larger.

Politely decline further servings.

Keep meal servings to one scoop or dish or less when assembling your plate.

Food Management Everyday
Change your eating routine to one that you won't associate with food.
Before eating anything you are desiring, wait 20 minutes.

Before you eat, down a big glass of water or diet Coke.

Keep a large glass or bottle of water nearby to sip on throughout the day.

Steer clear of high-calorie condiments like coffee cream, butter, mayonnaise, and salad dressings.
Shopping
Shop without being hungry or worn out.

Make a list before you go shopping, and don't buy anything from it.

If you must indulge in enticing meals, get single-serve packets and look for a lower-calorie substitute.

Do not sample products in the store.
Read the food labels. To assist you in making the healthiest decisions, compare goods.

Preparation
When preparing meals, chew some gum.

If you want to taste-test your food, use a quarter teaspoon.

Try to only prepare what you will eat so you won't have any leftovers.

If you've made more food than you need, divide it up into little containers and store them in the freezer or refrigerator right away.

Avoid eating while preparing meals.

Eating

Eat gradually. Keep in mind that it takes your stomach 20 minutes to signal your brain that it is full. Do not believe that you are hungry when you are not.

To eat properly, you should take a mouthful, set your utensil down, sip some water, cut your next bite, take a little, put your tool down, and so on.

Don't chop your food in one sitting. Only cut as necessary.

Eat slowly, and chew each bite thoroughly.

At least once throughout a meal or snack, put your fork down for a minute or two.

Take pauses to think and chat with others.

Cleanup and Remaining Food

Label leftovers with the meal or snack they belong to.

Keep leftovers in little pieces in the refrigerator or freezer.
If you are still hungry, don't tidy.

Social and out-of-home dining
Avoid showing up hungry. Before the meal, eat something small.

Eat plenty of low-calorie items, such as fruits and vegetables, and consume lesser amounts of high-calorie meals.
eat the foods you enjoy, but only in moderation.

Wait at least 20 minutes after a meal before deciding whether you want seconds or whether your eyes are bigger than your stomach.

Limit your alcohol consumption. Try lime-flavored soda water. To preserve space for the big occasion, don't skip any of the day's other meals.

When dining

Order off the menu rather than from the buffet.

Instead of bread, ask for some veggies or a salad as an appetizer.

Share high-calorie dishes with someone if you order them.

Attempt a mint with your coffee after supper.
 If you do have dessert, split it between two or more individuals.

Avoid overeating if you want to avoid wasting food.
To bring additional food home, request a doggy bag.

Before the meal is given to you, request that the waitress place half of your entree in a to-go bag.
Request high-fat sauces, gravy, or salad dressing on the side.

 Before each bite, dab the fork tip in the dressing.

If bread is offered, request only one slice.

Try it without any oil or butter.

Use a little amount of oil and a lot of vinegar for dipping when ordering bread at Italian restaurants that provide oil and vinegar.

In a Friend's Residence

Bring a low-calorie entrée, appetizer, or dessert if you can.

Tell the host that you'll only be having a limited quantity or serve yourself tiny servings.

Get up or move away from the snack table. If you are near the food, stay away from the kitchen or keep occupied.

Reduce your alcohol consumption.

In cafeterias and buffets
Your plate should be mostly lettuce and/or veggies.

Instead of using a dinner plate, use a salad plate.
Dishes should be put away after a meal before drinking coffee or tea.

Having a Party at Home
Look at cookbooks with reduced cholesterol and fat.

Use single-serving meals like hamburger patties or chicken breasts.

Prepare sweets and appetizers with fewer calories.

Holidays
Keep all enticing foods hidden.

Create a home decoration without using food.

Prepare low-calorie snacks and drinks for visitors.

Permit one plan to treat every day for yourself.

To save money for the holiday feast, don't miss meals.
Eat scheduled, routine meals.

Possess a Positive Attitude

Make maintaining a healthy weight a top goal.

Be sensible. Instead of focusing on achieving the lowest weight or the optimum weight determined by calculations or tables, set an objective to get healthy.
Instead of dieting, emphasize a healthy eating pattern. Dieting often only lasts a short while and seldom results in long-term success.

Take a long view. You are creating new, healthy habits that you will adopt over the next month, a year, and a decade.

Chapter 2

Get free from binge eating

Disordered eating pattern
A significant eating condition called binge-eating disorder causes you to repeatedly eat unusually big amounts of food and feels you can't stop.

Everybody occasionally overeats, whether it's eating seconds or thirds of a festive feast. However, for some individuals, excessive overeating that spirals out of control and starts to happen often crosses the threshold into binge-eating disorder.

If you have a binge-eating disorder, you could feel ashamed of your excess and commit to stopping. But you feel such a strong compulsion that you are powerless to control your cravings and keep eating in excess.

Symptoms

You can be at a normal weight although most persons with binge-eating disorder are fat or overweight. The following are behavioral and emotional indicators of binge-eating disorder:

*Eating a disproportionately high amount of food in a short period, such as two hours

*Feeling as though your eating habits are fast deteriorating during binge episodes

*Eating till you're sated but not satisfied

*Eating alone or covertly a lot

*Feeling down about your eating, disgusted, humiliated, guilty, or upset

*Often dieting, maybe without seeing any weight reduction

You don't often compensate for extra calories consumed after a binge by vomiting, taking laxatives, or engaging in strenuous exercise, unlike a person with bulimia. You might try eating a diet or regular meals.

However, limiting your diet could just encourage more binge eating.

The frequency of binge events each week determines the severity of the binge-eating problem.

When to visit a doctor

As soon as you notice any binge-eating disorder signs, get in touch with a doctor. If untreated, binge eating disorders can range in duration from brief to recurring, or they can last for years.

Discuss your binge eating symptoms and sentiments with a medical practitioner or a mental health expert. If you're hesitant to get help, talk to a trusted friend or relative about how you're feeling. You can start the process of treating binge-eating disorder successfully with the assistance of a friend, family member, instructor, or religious leader.

Helping a family member with symptoms

and skilled at disguising their behavior, a person with a binge-eating disorder may make it challenging for others to see the issue.

Have an honest conversation with your loved one if you believe they may be experiencing binge-eating disorder symptoms.

Encourage and assist others.

Offer to assist your loved one in locating and scheduling an appointment with a licensed medical or mental health practitioner. You could even propose joining them.

Your chance of getting a binge-eating disorder may be affected by the following factors:

Family background.

If your parents or siblings have (or have had) an eating disorder, you are far more likely to as well. This may suggest that the chance of having an eating disorder is increased by inherited genes.

Dieting. There is a history of dieting among many persons who have binge eating disorders. In particular, if you are experiencing signs of sadness, dieting or reducing calories during the day may make you feel the want to binge eat.

Psychiatric problems: Binge eaters frequently have unfavorable self-perceptions of their abilities and accomplishments. Stress, a negative body image, and the availability of favorite binge foods can all be triggers for binging.

Complications

You could have physical and mental side effects from binge eating.

The following are complications that may result from binge eating disorder:

A low standard of living:

Functional issues in your personal life, at business, or in social circumstances
social exclusion

Obesity

Obesity-associated illnesses such as joint issues, heart disease, type 2 diabetes, gastroesophageal reflux disease (GERD), and various respiratory abnormalities that are connected to sleep

The following psychiatric conditions are frequently connected to binge-eating disorder:

Depression

Bipolar illness

Anxiety

diseases caused by drug usage

Prevention

Although there is no surefire technique to stop binge eating disorders if you exhibit binge eating symptoms, get expert assistance. Your healthcare professional can provide you with advice on where to turn for assistance.

Before things become worse, help a friend or loved one who you suspect has a binge-eating issue move toward healthy habits and get professional help.

If you are a parent:
Encourage and support positive body image, regardless of body type or size.
Talk about any worries you have with your child's primary care physician, who may be in a position to see early signs of an eating disorder and prevent its emergence.

Chapter 3

Intermittent fasting

Intermittent fasting: Is skipping meals a terrible idea or a secret weapon for losing weight? Intermittent fasting is one diet fad that doesn't seem to be going anywhere anytime soon. You do it when you consciously fast for a set period from eating or drinking anything but water. While some people fast for religious reasons, others do so to lose weight.

But is weight loss with intermittent fasting a healthy practice?

Can you get healthier by fasting intermittently?

Intermittent fasting for weight loss may provide some short-term advantages, according to recent studies.

It appears that short-term fasting can result in ketosis, a metabolic state in which the body burns down stored fat for energy when there is insufficient glucose available to do so. Ketone-like compounds grow as a result of this. This can result in weight reduction along with consuming fewer calories overall. According to research, alternate-day fasting is comparable to a standard low-calorie diet for weight loss.

Additionally, fasting has an impact on the body's metabolic functions, which may help to enhance blood sugar control, reduce inflammation, and increase the body's ability to respond to physical stress. According to some studies, this may help with inflammatory diseases including multiple sclerosis, asthma, and arthritis.

There hasn't been much long-term study on intermittent fasting to see how it impacts people over time. There are therefore no documented long-term health advantages or dangers.

Consequences of sporadic fasting
Unpleasant side effects might result from intermittent fasting. They could consist of nausea, constipation, headaches, lethargy, sleeplessness, irritability, poor attention,

and appetite. Most adverse effects disappear within a month.

Some people may find it simpler to maintain an intermittent fasting schedule than it is to track their calories every day. Others, particularly those with hectic or unpredictable schedules, find it harder to stick to an intermittent fasting plan.

Are you a candidate for intermittent fasting? Many people find intermittent fasting to be safe, but not everyone does.

For those who are under 18, have a history of disordered eating, are pregnant, or are nursing, skipping meals is not advised. It may be challenging for athletes to properly eat and replenish for an active lifestyle. Before beginning an intermittent fasting regimen, discuss with your medical team if you have diabetes or other health conditions.

Also, keep in mind that avoiding overeating during your meal windows is essential for successful weight reduction with intermittent fasting. Losing weight still relies on consuming fewer calories than you burn.

Getting the vitamins and minerals you require may be challenging if your eating window is reduced. It is crucial to consume meals when following this diet that is produced with high-quality, nutritious components, such as fruits, vegetables, whole grains, low-fat dairy, and lean protein.

If practiced too frequently, intermittent fasting might be harmful.

Dry fasting is a method that limits the amount of food and liquids consumed, which causes extreme dehydration and raises significant health issues. If the caloric restriction is too great, such as averaging less than 1,200 calories per day over time, malnutrition may result.

Chapter 4

Try Exercises

Limiting the number of calories consumed through food is one strategy that might assist someone in losing weight. The alternative is to increase calorie burn through exercise.

Advantages of exercise against diet

A healthier diet and regular exercise are both better for weight loss than calorie restriction alone.

Certain illnesses' consequences can be avoided or even reversed by exercise. Exercise reduces cholesterol and blood pressure, which may help to stave against a heart attack.

Additionally, exercising reduces your chance of getting some malignancies, like colon and breast cancer. Exercise is also known to support feelings of confidence and wellbeing, perhaps reducing anxiety and depressive symptoms.

Exercise aids in weight reduction and weight maintenance. Exercise can boost metabolism, which is the number of calories you burn each day. Lean body mass may be maintained and increased, which also contributes to a daily calorie burn rise.

How Much Exercise Is Required to Lose Weight?

It is advised that you engage in some type of aerobic exercise at least three times a week for a minimum of 20 minutes per session if you want to benefit from exercise's health benefits. If you want to genuinely reduce weight, it's best to exercise for longer than 20 minutes.

A daily regimen of just 15 minutes of moderate activity, such as walking a mile, can result in a 100-calorie calorie burn (provided you don't eat too many calories afterwards). For a year, burning 700 calories each week can result in a weight reduction of up to 10 pounds.

How to Determine Your Goal Heart Rate

You must mix in some higher-intensity workouts if you want to reap the full range of health advantages from exercise.

You may measure your heart rate to determine how hard you are working. The simplest method for calculating your desired heart rate is to remove your age from 220, and then divide that result by 60 to 80 per cent.

To find your ideal intensity for each workout, see a trainer or your medical team. Before starting any fitness program, anyone with unique health problems like an injury, diabetes, or heart disease should speak with a doctor.

It doesn't matter what kind of exercise you perform to lose weight as much as if you do it at all. For this reason, experts advise choosing exercises you love to maintain a regular schedule.

Aerobic

Whatever fitness regimen you choose to follow should contain some sort of aerobic or cardiovascular activity. Exercises that are aerobic increase heart rate and blood circulation. Aerobic exercises include cycling, swimming, dancing, walking, and running. You can exercise with a fitness machine like a stair stepper, elliptical, or treadmill.

Strength Training

Gaining muscle when exercising with weights has several benefits, including helping you lose fat. In turn, muscle burns calories. What a positive feedback cycle!

Making Exercise a Part of Your Lifestyle

More important than whether or not you exercise in a particular session is the overall quantity of activity you get in a day. Because of this, even little adjustments to your everyday routine can have a significant impact on your waistline.

Following a healthy lifestyle includes the following:

Before You Begin an Exercise Program, consider walking or riding your bike to work or while running errands, choosing the stairs over the elevator, parking further away from destinations, and walking the remaining distance.
Before beginning a new fitness regimen, especially if you want to engage in severe activity, see your doctor. This is particularly crucial if you have:

Heart condition
lung condition
Diabetes
kidney illness
Arthritis
Before beginning a new fitness regimen, those who have been particularly inactive

lately, are overweight or have recently quit smoking should also see their doctors.

It's crucial to pay attention to your body's cues when you initially begin a new fitness regimen. You should exert more effort so that your level of fitness increases. However, straining oneself beyond your limits might lead to harm. If you begin to feel discomfort or become breathless, stop exercising.

Chapter 5

Avoid this extreme:Anorexia

Anorexia is an eating disorder that is distinguished by unusually low body weight, a strong fear of gaining weight, and a skewed sense of weight. People with anorexia put great emphasis on maintaining their weight and form, making excessive attempts that frequently seriously disrupt their lives.

The amount of food consumed by anorexics is typically highly restricted to avoid weight gain or to keep dropping weight. By utilizing laxatives, diet supplements, diuretics, or enemas improperly, they might reduce their caloric intake by throwing up just after eating. Additionally, they could try to shed weight by overexerting themselves. The person's worry about weight gain persists despite weight loss.

It's not really about eating with anorexia. Trying to deal with emotional issues in this way is very harmful and can even be fatal. Being thin is frequently associated with self-worth when you have anorexia.

Like other eating disorders, anorexia may have a serious impact on your life and be very challenging to treat. However, with therapy, you may regain a stronger sense of who you are, return to healthier eating patterns, and undo some of the worst side effects of anorexia.

Symptoms

Starvation is a factor in the physical manifestations of anorexia nervosa. An inaccurate sense of body weight and an extraordinarily potent fear of gaining weight or being fat are additional emotional and behavioral problems associated with anorexia.

Given that everyone's definition of low body weight is varied and that some people may not appear to be exceedingly thin, it may be challenging to identify the signs and symptoms. Additionally, those who suffer from anorexia frequently hide their physical issues, eating patterns, or thinness.

Bodily symptoms
The following are examples of anorexia's physical symptoms:

Extreme weight loss or failure to attain the anticipated weight throughout the development
Unusual blood counts and a thin look
Fatigue
Insomnia
nausea or fainting
fingers with bluish discolouration
thinning, broken, or missing hair
Lack of menstruation Soft, downy hair covering the body
stomach discomfort and diarrhea

Yellowish or dry skin
dislike of the cold
irregular heartbeat
minimal blood pressure
Dehydration
Arms or legs swelling
Forced vomiting resulted in eroded teeth and calluses on the knuckles.
Some anorexics engage in binge-and-purge behavior, much like bulimics. However, those who struggle with anorexia frequently have abnormally low body weights, whereas those who suffer from bulimia frequently have normal to above-normal weights.

Symptoms of the mind and behavior
Anorexic behavior may involve attempting to reduce weight by:

severely limiting one's food intake via fasting or dieting
overtraining in exercise

Using laxatives, enemas, diet aids, or herbal medicines, among other methods, to cause vomiting and binge-eating to get rid of food
The following are examples of emotional and behavioral symptoms:

obsession with food, which occasionally involves preparing extravagant meals for others but not consuming them.
often missing or refusing to eat meals
denial of hunger or providing justifications for not eating
consuming just a certain number of "safe" meals, often ones that are low in fat and calories
adopting strict eating or eating-related habits, such as throwing out food after chewing
avoiding eating in front of others
falsifying the amount of food consumed
Fear of gaining weight, which may involve often weighing or measuring one's body or frequently inspecting one's reflection for any perceived defects

complaining about one's weight or the presence of certain bodily components
putting on many layers of clothes
No emotion (lack of emotion)
social exclusion
Irritability
Insomnia
less desire for sex
when to visit the doctor
Unfortunately, a large majority of anorexics first reject therapy. Their health is less important than their desire to maintain their thinness. Insist that your loved one see a doctor if you have any concerns about them.

Get assistance if you're dealing with any of the aforementioned issues or believe you may have an eating disorder. Try to find a confidant with whom you can discuss your anorexia if you're keeping it from close ones.

Causes

Anorexia has an elusive specific aetiology. Similar to many illnesses, it most likely results from a confluence of biological, psychological, and environmental variables.

Biological. There may be genetic abnormalities that put certain people at a higher risk of developing anorexia, while it is not yet known which genes are implicated. Perfectionism, sensitivity, and persistence are characteristics linked to anorexia and may be inherited in certain people.

Psychological. Some anorexics may have obsessive-compulsive personality characteristics that make it simpler to follow rigid diets and avoid eating even when they are hungry. They could have a severe obsession with perfection, which makes them believe they're never skinny enough. Additionally, they might be extremely anxious and turn to restrict eating to calm themselves.

Environmental.Thinness is valued in contemporary Western society. Success and value are frequently connected with physical attractiveness.

Especially among young girls, peer pressure may contribute to the desire to be skinny.

danger signs

In girls and women, anorexia is more prevalent.However, eating disorders are rapidly becoming a problem for boys and men, maybe as a result of mounting social pressure.

Teenagers are more likely than adults to have anorexia. Even so, it's uncommon in those over 40, though it can happen to anyone at any age. Teenagers may be particularly vulnerable because of all the changes that occur throughout puberty to their bodies.

Additionally, they could experience more peer pressure and be more sensitive to judgment or even innocuous remarks about their weight or body type.

Anorexia is made more likely by several circumstances, such as:

Genetics. A person's chance of developing anorexia may increase if certain genes are altered. A person is far more likely to develop anorexia if they have a first-degree family who did, such as a parent, sibling, or kid.

Hunger and dieting. Dieting increases the likelihood of having an eating disorder. There is compelling evidence that many anorexia symptoms are true signs of malnutrition. The effects of starvation on the brain include changes in mood, rigidity in thought, anxiety, and decreased appetite. Starvation and weight loss may alter how the brain functions in susceptible people, which might lead to the perpetuation of restrictive eating practices and make it challenging to resume regular eating habits.

Transitions. Change can cause mental stress and raise the risk of anorexia, whether it's a new school, house, or work; the end of a relationship; or the loss or sickness of a loved one.

Complications

Numerous issues can arise from anorexia. It can be deadly if it's severe enough. Even when a person is not very underweight, death can strike without warning. This might be brought on by irregular cardiac rhythms (arrhythmias) or an electrolyte imbalance—a deficiency in the minerals sodium, potassium, and calcium, which keep the fluid balance in your body—in your body.

Anorexia also has other side effects, such as:

Anaemia

Heart issues such as mitral valve prolapse, irregular heartbeats, or heart failure

Osteoporosis, a loss of bone, increases the risk of fractures

Muscle wasting

Lack of menstruation in women

lower testosterone levels in men
gastrointestinal issues such as bloating, nausea, or constipation
anomalies in electrolytes, including low blood potassium, sodium, and chloride levels
a kidney condition
Every organ in the body, including the brain, heart, and kidneys, can suffer harm in a severely malnourished anorexic. Even when anorexia is in check, this harm might not entirely be repairable.

People with anorexia frequently also have various mental health concerns in addition to a plethora of physical difficulties. They might consist of

Depression, anxiety, and other mental health issues
personality defects
Disorders of obsession and ritual
abuse of drugs and alcohol

Self-harm, suicidal ideas, or attempts at suicide

Prevention

There is no certain strategy to stave off anorexia nervosa. Primary care doctors (paediatricians, family doctors, and internists) may be in a strong position to see anorexia's early warning signs and stop the condition from becoming severe. During normal medical checkups, for instance, they might inquire about eating habits and contentment with looks.

Consider talking to a family member or acquaintance about these concerns if you observe that they are struggling with poor self-esteem, strict dietary routines, or body image difficulties. You can discuss better practices or available treatments even if you might not be able to stop an eating disorder from arising.

www.ingramcontent.com/pod-product-compliance
Lightning Source LLC
Chambersburg PA
CBHW072328270726
48658CB00016B/2129